The Menopause Whisper Network: A Quick Guide to Uncommon Symptoms

Dedicated to the women who dare to break the silence around menopause. This book is for you, with a special thanks to those whose online stories fueled my passion to share this knowledge.

No table of contents entries found.

Part 1: Introduction

Perimenopause: A Confusing Journey, But You're Not Alone

Turning 45, my body started to change in unexpected ways. Digestive issues, aches, and pains became my new normal. Already prone to anxiety, it intensified, impacting my well-being. Doctor visits and tests became frequent, but everything came back normal. The literature focused heavily on hot flashes, but many of my symptoms weren't addressed. Confusion and fear took hold. Was this the beginning of a serious illness?

Slowly but surely, my familiar body felt foreign. Emotions simmered just below the surface, and physical sensations were magnified. Pain became a constant presence. Aches and discomfort settled in my shoulders, back, and jaw, to name a few. Weight gain was gradual and constant.
The emotional impact mirrored the physical. Vulnerability became a constant companion, tears welling up easily, and frustration flaring unexpectedly. The isolation, however, was the sharpest pang. I felt like I was traversing this strange land entirely alone.

Searching for answers and trying to find some relief, I consulted doctors, friends, and family, but no one seemed to understand. Driven by desperation, I dove into on-line research and books. Most resources painted an incomplete picture, listing only a few symptoms. My reality felt entirely different.

Finally, online chat groups offered a lifeline. Reading about other women's experiences, it hit me – they weren't sure either, just like me! They questioned whether their symptoms were normal and sought advice on managing them. Tears streamed down my face – happy tears this time. I wasn't alone! There were other women with the same strange symptoms, searching for answers and supporting each other.

These online communities became my source of support. Women openly shared stories, fears, and coping strategies. It was a wealth of information not found in any book. Inspired by this sisterhood, I decided to write this book – a raw, unfiltered look at menopause experiences.
Listen, I'm not a doctor nor a scientist. I'm just a regular woman who went on a wild goose chase to figure out what was happening to me. I don't claim to have all the answers about menopause, not by a long shot. But what I do have is my story, and some online chats that were a lifesaver for me.

So this book is not a medical guide. It's about the diversity, strangeness, and suddenness of perimenopause symptoms. My goal is to help women understand they're not alone.
Here I am, ten years later, and feeling much better. The intensity, frequency, and strangeness of symptoms have subsided. I learned there are good

and bad days, with no miracle solution. However, the most important lesson was the power of knowledge. Just knowing these symptoms were likely hormonal fluctuations, not a disease, eased my fears and anxiety, and allowed me to look in the right places for relief.

This newfound understanding not only helped me accept the bad days, but also brought a sense of serenity. It wasn't a death sentence, just a natural transition. This empowered me to accept these challenging years with an increased serenity.

What was the most surprising to me is that in this age of information, women still struggle to find answers about menopause. After all, half the world's population goes through this change! Why wasn't more information readily available about the multitude of symptoms? Why wasn't there more research on this topic?

For generations, menopause has been a taboo subject. For some reason, it's not a subject that comes up naturally even among women. This secrecy has left women feeling like they're going through a personal apocalypse, alone!

But I feel that a positive change is emerging! Celebrities are stepping out and sharing their menopause journeys. By openly discussing these natural transitions, they're chipping away at the stigma. It's a cultural power move, sparking a collective consciousness and letting women know they're not alone.

It's time to shed light on this essential chapter in a woman's life and empower her to navigate it with confidence and a newfound sense of sisterhood. In this book, I'll share some of my own symptoms and experiences, along with unfiltered voices from the online communities that became my lifeline. Together, let's break the silence and empower ourselves. Let's make this next chapter a better-lit walk, not a confusing journey!

Lifting the Lid on Menopause: What it is, When it Hits, and Why You're Not Crazy

Ah, menopause. The mere mention of it can spark a chorus of groans and knowing glances. Hot flashes, mood swings, the end of an era – these are just some of the images conjured by this natural transition. But what exactly is menopause, and why does it happen to us? Buckle up, because in this chapter, we'll shed some light on this biological shift, debunk some myths, and offer a resounding truth: you're not crazy, you're simply going through menopause!

What is Menopause?

In its most basic definition, menopause, according to the National Institute on Aging, is the permanent cessation of menstruation. It marks the official end of a woman's reproductive years and typically occurs between the ages of 45 and 55. However, there's some wiggle room here – menopause can happen earlier or later depending on individual factors.

Perimenopause

Think of menopause as the grand finale, but before the curtain falls, there's a whole act dedicated to setting the stage. This introductory act is called perimenopause, a transitional phase that can last anywhere from a few years to a decade. During this time, your body's symphony conductor – the hormones – starts playing a slightly off-key tune.

Estrogen and progesterone production fluctuates, leading to a variety of symptoms that can leave you feeling like you're in a musical out of sync.

Now, before you start picturing menopause as a symphony of woes, here's a bright note: It's a natural process, and it doesn't have to define you! Many women experience relief from some pre-menopausal symptoms, such as PMS. Menopause can also be a time of personal growth and empowerment – a chance to rediscover yourself and embrace a new chapter in your life.

Let's delve into the key players in this hormonal orchestra: estrogen, progesterone, and testosterone, and explore how their fluctuating levels during perimenopause impact your wellbeing.

Estrogen

Estrogen, often referred to as the "female hormone," is a group of hormones with several crucial roles in your body. During your reproductive years, estrogen keeps your menstrual cycle running like clockwork. It regulates the thickening of the uterine lining in preparation for pregnancy, stimulates ovulation, and influences vaginal lubrication. But as you enter perimenopause, estrogen production by your ovaries starts to wane. This decline is gradual at first, but it can accelerate in the years leading up to menopause.

Progesterone

Progesterone works hand-in-hand with estrogen to orchestrate your menstrual cycle. It helps prepare the uterine lining for a fertilized egg and plays a vital role in maintaining a healthy pregnancy. However, just like estrogen, progesterone production also starts to decline during perimenopause. This decline disrupts the delicate balance between estrogen and progesterone, leading to unpredictable menstrual cycles and other symptoms.

Testosterone

Testosterone, often thought of as a male hormone, also plays a role in women's health. It contributes to bone health, muscle mass, and libido. While testosterone levels naturally decline with age in both men and women, some women may experience a relative increase in testosterone compared to the declining estrogen levels during perimenopause. This can lead to symptoms like increased facial hair or acne.

A Rundown of Common and Uncommon Menopause Symptoms

Menopause is associated in a big way to hot flashes, the most notorious symptom associated with this transition. But menopause is more than just feeling like a human furnace. It's a symphony of changes orchestrated by your body, and sometimes, the instruments go a little out of tune, leading to a variety of symptoms, both common and uncommon. Let's delve into the flames and explore the diverse experiences women face during menopause.

Common and Uncommon Menopause Symptoms

While some symptoms take center stage during menopause, others play more subtle roles. Here are some experiences that women might encounter:

- Hot flashes – those sudden bursts of heat that leave you feeling like you've stepped out of a sauna – are a hallmark symptom of menopause. They can strike at any time, day or night, and can be accompanied by sweating, chills, and a rapid heartbeat.
- Your once-reliable menstrual cycle goes rogue, with periods becoming irregular, heavier, lighter, or even disappearing altogether. This unpredictability can be frustrating and stressful.
- Difficulty falling asleep, staying asleep, or waking up frequently at night can leave you feeling exhausted and foggy-brained. Sleep disturbances are a common complaint during menopause.
- Hormonal fluctuations can trigger a rollercoaster of emotions, leading to irritability, mood swings, and anxiety. You might feel like you're on a hair-trigger, and even small things can set you off.
- Brain fog, characterized by forgetfulness, difficulty concentrating, and mental haziness, can be a frustrating symptom of menopause. It can feel like your brain is stuck in a thick fog, making it hard to focus on tasks or remember things.
- Vaginal dryness can make sex uncomfortable and increase your risk of

urinary tract infections. This can negatively impact your sex life and intimacy with your partner.
- Weight gain, particularly around the middle, due to hormonal changes, especially a decrease in estrogen, can lead to the body storing more fat around the abdomen.
- Heart palpitations, a sudden feeling like your heart is racing or skipping a beat, can be a startling symptom of menopause.
- Increased joint pain and stiffness can be a new reality for some women.
- Bloating, gas, and changes in bowel habits are not uncommon.
- Hair loss and thinning can be a concern for some women.
- Tingling sensations and internal vibrations can happen.

What is special about menopause is that it's a highly individual experience. You might experience all, some, or none of the symptoms listed above. The intensity and duration of these symptoms can also vary greatly from woman to woman.

Pain and Hormone Fluctuation During Menopause

Menopause brings a cascade of hormonal changes. Estrogen and progesterone see significant declines during this transition. This decline is linked to various symptoms experienced by women, including pain. Let's delve into the science behind this connection:

The Role of Estrogen

- **Estrogen and Inflammation:** Estrogen has anti-inflammatory properties. As estrogen levels drop during menopause, the body's inflammatory response can become heightened. This increased inflammation is believed to contribute to various types of pain experienced by women in menopause.
- **Musculoskeletal Pain:** Estrogen plays a role in maintaining bone health and muscle strength. Declining estrogen levels can contribute to joint pain, muscle stiffness, and an increased risk of osteoarthritis.
- **Headaches:** Fluctuations in estrogen levels are linked to migraines, especially in women with a history of migraines before menopause.

Additional Considerations

- **Central Nervous System:** The central nervous system plays a crucial role in pain perception. Menopause can affect brain chemistry, potentially leading to increased pain sensitivity.
- **Psychological Factors:** Anxiety and depression, which are more common during menopause, can influence how women perceive and experience pain.

Further Research

The exact mechanisms by which hormonal changes during menopause lead to pain are still being explored. Researchers are investigating the complex interplay between hormones, the nervous system, and other factors in influencing pain perception during this life stage.

Traditional and Natural Treatments for Menopause Symptoms

This chapter will explore both traditional and natural treatment options to help you manage your symptoms.

Traditional Therapies

Western medicine offers a variety of tools to manage menopause symptoms. Here's a look at some of the most common options:

- **Hormone Replacement Therapy (HRT):** HRT is often the first line of defense, aiming to replace the declining levels of estrogen and progesterone. It can come in various forms, such as pills, patches, creams, or gels. HRT can be very effective in alleviating hot flashes, night sweats, vaginal dryness, and mood swings. However, it's important to discuss the potential risks and benefits with your doctor to see if it's the right choice for you.
- **Low-Dose Antidepressants:** For some women, low-dose antidepressants can be helpful in managing symptoms like mood swings, anxiety, and sleep problems. These medications work by increasing the levels of certain neurotransmitters in the brain that can be impacted by hormonal fluctuations.
- **Prescription Sleep Aids:** If sleep disturbances are a major concern, your doctor might prescribe sleep medications to help you fall asleep and stay asleep. However, these medications should be used

cautiously and for short periods to avoid dependence.

Natural Allies

Traditional medicine isn't the only weapon in your arsenal. Nature provides a bounty of options to help manage menopause symptoms:

- **Lifestyle Changes:** Simple adjustments to your daily routine can make a big difference. Regular exercise, stress management techniques like yoga or meditation, and a healthy diet rich in fruits, vegetables, and whole grains can all contribute to reducing symptoms and improving overall well-being.
- **Herbal Remedies:** Black cohosh, red clover, and evening primrose oil are some popular herbal supplements used to manage hot flashes and other menopause symptoms. However, it's important to talk to your doctor before starting any herbal remedies, as they can interact with other medications.
- **Dietary Supplements:** Certain vitamins and minerals, such as vitamin D, calcium, and magnesium, can be helpful in managing symptoms like bone loss, sleep disturbances, and mood swings. Discuss with your doctor if supplementation is right for you based on any deficiencies you might have.

- **Mindfulness and meditation:** These relaxing practices might not be magic bullets, but they can be a helpful toolbox. Think of it like this: mindfulness helps you focus on what's happening right now, not freaking out about the future or reliving the past. That can take the edge off that pesky anxiety that loves to show up during this hormonal shift. Plus, a calmer mind can sometimes lead to a better night's sleep (no promises on night sweats, though). Meditation can even be a way to deal with aches and pains – it teaches you to acknowledge them without getting all worked up about them.

So, if you're feeling overwhelmed, find a quiet corner, take a few deep breaths, and give mindfulness a try. It might not be a cure-all, but it could be a helpful addition to your menopause survival kit.

Bioidentical Hormones and the WHI Study

In the 1990s, bioidentical hormone therapy (BHRT) emerged as an alternative to traditional hormone replacement therapy (HRT) for managing menopause. Both approaches aim to ease symptoms by introducing hormones back into the body. However, BHRT uses plant-derived hormones (often soy or yam) that are chemically similar to those our bodies naturally produce. Traditional HRT, on the other hand, utilizes synthetic hormones with slightly different structures. Proponents of BHRT believe this closer match translates to fewer side effects and improved symptom relief for some women, although research hasn't definitively proven this.

In the 1980s, a large study called the Women's Health Initiative (WHI) raised concerns about an increased risk of breast cancer with some forms of HRT. This study had a significant impact on how HRT was prescribed, leading many women to avoid it altogether. However, further research and analysis of the WHI data revealed some important nuances. The increased risk was found primarily in women who started HRT many years after menopause, and the absolute risk increase was relatively small. Additionally, the WHI study used a specific combination of hormones (conjugated equine estrogen and progestin) that may not be the best choice for all women.

Today, with a more comprehensive understanding of HRT, doctors can tailor treatment plans using different types and delivery methods of hormones to minimize potential risks. If you're considering HRT or BHRT, it's important to discuss the latest research and your individual risk factors with your doctor to make an informed decision.

Part 2: The Voices of the Whisper Network

In the next chapter, I'll share some of the most helpful posts I've found online during my search for answers about menopause. I've been scouring online communities, and I want to pass on what I've learned. It's been a challenging journey, one of the most difficult I've faced, and these posts have been a valuable resource. My goal is to share the knowledge and support I found with others going through this transition.

Body Betrayed: When Hot Flashes Are More Than Just Heat

I started experiencing a series of uncomfortable episodes throughout the day. My heart rate would increase, followed by a subtle headache and nausea. There was a general feeling of unease, and then a distinct warming sensation in my chest and face. These weren't exactly the dramatic hot flashes I'd seen portrayed in movies and on social media. The experience was more complex and involved a range of symptoms.

So forget the stereotype of just feeling warm! The following posts showcase the diverse and unexpected symptoms women experience with hot flashes. Dive in and see just how different each woman's journey can be.

"Do any of you feel really nauseated with your hot flashes? Mine seem to be increasing in intensity. I've tried all the tricks to at least reducing the symptoms and I'm not having much luck. Exercising, cutting down sugar, not eating spicy foods, drinking plenty of water. I also have vertigo issues that have intensified with it, have had that my whole life but definitely has increased and gotten worse with this. I hope this doesn't last forever."

"Good Morning! I'm having extreme hot flashes which then causes me to panic and then my blood

pressure goes up I've never had high BP before I go to the Drs today and I was wondering if anyone has dealt with this I'm hoping if he can help control the hot flashes I won't need any BP medication but these panic attacks are the worse I feel loss and I've been to the ER 4 times in 3 weeks bc I have these episodes I can feel the hot flashes followed by high BP then my panic sits in....I can not keep doing this. Thank you for reading this, any input is greatly appreciated."

"Has anyone had a hot flash that caused them to faint? I woke up the other night from a hot flash and felt really woozy. I went into the bathroom to run cold water over my wrists and next thing I knew I was waking up on the tile floor. Pretty sure I caught myself with my face. Lol. I've read that hot flashes can cause dizziness but wasn't sure how common it is to actually faint."

"Ok so, hot flashes talk.... I'm not having defined hot flashes, I'm having little waves of "Woo I'm feeling a little warm all of a sudden" then dies down, ALL! DAY! LONG! Sitting at the computer, doing the dishes, going pee, doesn't matter what I'm doing or not doing... and it's ALL! NIGHT! LONG too! So, as you may guess, I'm not sleeping because of it! When my grown adult child hugged me during one of my little warm waves, they commented that I felt feverish. They could feel my heat, but my thermometer is telling me I'm "normal"! And I am not sick! Anyone else with this? WTF?!!!! "

"Talk to me about hot flashes ! Initially it was my chest and back mainly when I was sleeping. Now it's 3-5 minutes of full body sweat…feet and legs included and also happens during the day! I sometimes wake up and have to change all my clothes including underwear. The flipside of that is chills right before or right after the hot flash. Are these indeed hot flashes ??"

The Shivering Spell: Exploring the Mystery of Menopausal Chills

An unsettling chill would settle over me, not just a general coolness, but a deep full body cold or a more targeted one in my hands and feet. No matter how hard I tried, nothing could chase it away. Hot showers, usually a haven of warmth, offered no relief. These episodes of intense cold would come and go unpredictably, leaving me feeling like a thermostat malfunctioning within my own body. The strangest part was the prickling sensation, like pins and needles, that sometimes attacked my feet when the hot water hit them. It was a bizarre and frightening experience.

Then, I came across some posts shared by others. Reading about similar experiences lessened my fear. It turns out, these unexpected chills and strange sensations might not be as uncommon as I thought.

"I have a question about feeling cold.

I'm always so cold, my hands, legs, and my whole body freezing. I am waiting for blood tests around my thyroid. However this is ridiculous, I'm on HRT usually pretty warm, not anymore I'm absolutely freezing , any suggestions until i get my results on Thursday ???? and I've tried warm baths, showers, heat bags and more clothes. It doesn't matter if I'm still cold. less clothing and blankets.. I am just at a loss??? thank you for your answers and support"

"So, anyone suffering from low body temperature. When I take my temperature it's around 96. Yesterday I was feeling cold after dinner, when I finally began warming up my fingers and toes began to feel like frostbite. I also noticed after one of these episodes that if I try to throw warm water on my hands it burns. I know this happens in cold weather, but at home?"

"Does anyone feel cold all the time no matter what the weather is like? Apart from the hot flushes the rest of the time I'm freezing I've had had blood tests done for anemia and B12 they were fine"

*"Last night I was actually COLD for the first time in YEARS!! I was so cold I slept in a hoodie cuddle close to my man for warmth. He asked if I was feeling ok because I am NEVER cold.
I was even cold this morning!! Am I through menopause?!?
It felt good wearing a hoodie and not sweating to death*

I'm ok with cold "

"Ha! Menopause cold flashes are a thing! Who knew? Anyone else suffering from muscle cramps as a result of feeling cold? I've had this for two years. The pain from the cramps makes me literally cry (tears) and it wakes me out of my sleep sometimes. I tried a magnesium, potassium & zinc vitamin, along with calcium, and it didn't help. Not even a little. I can feel warm/hot on my torso because of the environment I'm in and have icicle fingers. It's torture. I work in a courtroom with a judge who gets hot easily so he cranks the AC. I'm literally the only person in the courtroom who cannot hide my hands for warmth. I can't refuse to work with him. I don't know what to do. I'm so tired of being unhappy."

Unbearable Joint Pain? It Might Be Menopause, Not Disease

Picture this: you're a fitness enthusiast – yoga, walks, dance nights, you name it. Then, BAM! This mystery pain creeps in, starting with your hands and fingers, then elbows, knees, hips – all join the party, leaving you feeling achy all over. Stairs become mini-mountains, opening jars requires the grip strength of a superhero, and suddenly you feel decades older than your actual age. It's enough to make anyone scared and frustrated, right? That was me and the surprise attack of menopausal joint pain. They say misery loves company, so let's just say the anti-inflammatory meds and muscle relaxers became my new BFFs in the battle against the aches.

Ever feel like your doctor doesn't quite get the whole "menopause body aches" thing? You're not alone. These social media posts showcase just how widespread this struggle is, despite the lack of attention it often receives.

"Hello everyone, I believe I'm in perimenopause, despite what my doctor thinks. Since September, I've been experiencing increasingly severe pain (back, shoulders, neck... joints... muscle pain, even in my arms...). I also have crying spells, irritability, and periods every 15 days! So, I've been taking St. John's wort since January, magnesium for as long as I can remember, and I went to the doctor. The blood tests didn't show anything, so he thinks it's arthritis

and has prescribed me chondroitin and glucosamine for the past few days. I've changed my mattress and pillow, I've seen a chiropractor, but nothing has worked. My husband tells me to stop looking and just accept that I'm in perimenopause."

"My joint pain is unbearable. Any suggestions I went to dr said I have degenerative disc disease and arthritis. Taking turmeric, doing PT, cbd cream, massages, thc cream, advil, Tylenol, baths nothing seems to be working I am thinking of going on BHRT or doing acupuncture or chiropractor- anything help you ladies out there."

"Been in awful joint and muscle pain for months and today was the worst , so I made the call to the doctor about going on HRT(first available appointment 28th sept) .. has anybody had any improvement with joint pain after going on HRT .. I'm doing what I can with weight loss and exercise but it's like one vicious circle"

"Hi everyone! I just wanted to introduce myself and say HI!!!!! I have been suffering with perimenopause joint pain for a while now but just confirmed with blood work that I am indeed in the thick of it. I don't want to take HRT and since I have had unusually severe and lengthy menstrual cycles my ferritin dropped to 7 so I have been exhausted. Good times!! Aging is not for sissies! Relieved and happy to be with other women going through similar issues and *hope to learn from your experiences and wisdom. Blessings to all.”*

“Do any women experience increased joint pain since peri/menopause? My knees pop and crack, finger joint pain and popping, elbows popping and shoulders popping along with joint pain. Body aches in places that I forgot even existed… not trying to sound whiny or complaining, just trying to make sense out of changes in my body that I'm experiencing. Big changes are taking place within my body and I'm concerned. Just helps to know that others have or are experiencing the same.”

The Body Buzz: The Weird Side Effects of Menopause

On top of the already disruptive menopause symptoms, a new wave of strangeness washed over me – internal tremors. These weren't full-body shakes, but a disorienting buzz that seemed to vibrate from deep within. It was an unsettling, almost scary sensation. My mind raced with possibilities, conjuring images of lurking diseases and the need for a complete medical workup. Just as anxiety began to tighten its grip, I stumbled upon these posts...

"I've seen many of you talk about feeling body tremors and some of you mention a creepy crawling sensation. What I feel is a sensation similar to restless legs but through my whole body. Is that like what you are feeling as well? It's driving me crazy!"

"Hi Ladies,has anyone experienced or are experiencing any Internal tremors/vibrations?For about 2 weeks now I am having Internal vibrations, sometimes in my head too,mostly at nights when you lay down and the body is in resting mode,also sometimes I get a headache with nausea together with the internal vibration.I had a CT SCAN ,came back normal,blood work normal for the most part,waiting on Thyroid result,The Doc said sometimes over active Thyroid can cause the tenors,I am 52 and never had any kind of Thyroid problems before.This situation makes me so

anxious, feels anxiety quickly,also I feel lightheaded at times,and sometimes feels like I can hear loud noise .Please let me know if anyone experiencing this.Thanks"

"I've read in posts here about internal vibrations. I call it feeling shaking, or off balance inside. My hands do not tremor, for example, so it's inside my body core. From my belly to my head. If I close my eyes I feel like I could topple over, like when I close my eyes to shampoo my hair. I have leaned against the shower to feel stable in those moments having my eyes closed. If I turned my head quickly to glance over my shoulder I felt almost dizzy, vertigo for a split second. Yesterday this sensation happened for a few hours. The internal "vibration" stopped first but instability remained a bit longer, then a slight headache and a kind of "Blah". Then it all went away. I don't remember any hot flashes during it but I had a couple afterward later in the day. Has anything like this happened to others?"

"Constant internal tremors, daily headaches, feeling off balance / lightheaded off and on every day and blurry vision…can all of these symptoms really be caused by menopause? Everything started completely out of the blue, all at once almost 2 years ago and I haven't been able to find any relief. I'm 48 and still have fairly regular cycles."

"Hello, I was wondering if anyone else suffers from very severe internal tremors or vibrations??? I have seen my doctors and specialists and they have no idea. It started slow here and there and then out of nowhere has become very severe. Mostly chest and abdo then goes down arms and legs. Feels like a constant racing vibration. Causes some tachycardia, eating makes it worse. No new medications when it started and bloods are all unremarkable. We were thinking I was peri earlier due to flushing, muscle and joint aches and pains and occasional low estrogen on bloods. I'm desperate for help as Drs can't help. Anyone else?"

The Body on Standby: A Dive into the Crippling Fatigue of Menopause

A wave of exhaustion unlike anything I'd ever known would suddenly wash over me. My limbs would feel heavy, as if weighted down by invisible anchors. Even the simplest tasks, like making a cup of coffee, felt like scaling a mountain. All I craved was the comfort of my bed, a desperate plea from my body for a seemingly endless slumber. This fatigue wasn't confined to specific times – it could strike anywhere, anytime. Like a thief, it stole my energy during a peaceful paddleboard session, leaving me stranded and needing help to shore. Feeling utterly defeated and lost, I stumbled upon these posts…

"My fatigue is debilitating. I can barely function. My doctor ran blood work and all of my levels are normal (thyroid, Vitamin D, B12, magnesium, etc). My FSH is in the postmenopausal range. HRT is NOT an option for me. Has anyone found any non-hormone solutions that have worked? I was exercising, but I can't even get through a moderate workout anymore. I'm now struggling to get through the work day and do simple things like fixing dinner and laundry. I may have my doc test me for hashimoto's since my sister does have it, but I seriously doubt that I do have it."

"My fatigue is bordering on a disability. Progesterone 200mg nightly along with Estrogen 0.75 patch. I know all of my symptoms contribute to fatigue. I had blood work for iron, Vit d, thyroid.. (all labs normal). I find it

hard to believe that menopause could make this much fatigue. Could the Progesterone linger all day.. Help!"

"I've never experienced fatigue like this. I'm sure my allergies add to it. I was told I may need allergy shots. I'm 3 years post menopause and most days fatigue is my constant companion. I can't work (at a desk job mind you) more than 4-5 hours. Then I come home and crash. I just forced myself to throw a load of laundry in the washer and cook dinner. Now I'm done. Anyone have this kind of fatigue?"

"Hi all, Has anyone ever had menopause cause fatigue so bad that you can barely even walk to the toilet and brain fog so severe that you can't hold a conversation, can't remember things (to the point I went to watch a comedian I love last week and can't remember anything). I also have no appetite at all. I wound up in hospital two weeks ago because my speech went really stuttery. I feel like my body and brain have just broken!
The doctor doesn't seem to know what's going on but has started me on HRT anyway!
Looking forward to hope that symptoms this severe can be normal and that it'll get better."

"Ladies, sometimes I get fatigued to the point that if I'm driving I need to pull over. It comes on suddenly and it lasts until I make myself get up and move. I'm literally struggling to keep my eyes open. It's a scary feeling, almost as if I'm drugged. Anyone else get

this? I've had tons of bloodwork and I've told my doctor many times, but never get an answer as to what's going on."

From Strong to Struggle: How Menopause Weakened My Muscles

On top of feeling tired all the time, my muscles seemed to give up too. My arms, legs, and hips felt weak. Even though I knew exercise would help, it felt impossible. Sometimes just walking was like dragging groceries around. Picking up groceries or opening doors became a struggle. I was so confused! Was this menopause too? Was I not eating enough protein or should I be exercising more? What was happening to my muscles? It was the strangest thing - some days I felt fine and could do everything normally, but other days I felt weak. Here's what other women shared about muscle weakness.

"Hello Lovely ladies! Does anyone experience muscle weakness? My muscles feel weak at times however, I can still lift and do things normally, it is just an odd feeling."

"I am a nervous wreck. I have been having random panic attacks, muscle weakness and tingling all over and a weird pressure in my head. I have not had a cycle since August of last year. Have any of you experienced these symptoms? I feel like I am losing my mind and fear something is seriously wrong with me. I went to the ER in December and had a CT, MRI and Eco and everything was good."

"Hello. Has anyone had constant muscle aches and weakness in arms and legs that lasted weeks? I went

in to do blood work and waited for results but my dr says menopause doesn't cause these symptoms but I have seen articles that claim differently."

"I have severe muscle weakness, anxiety, and fatigue that came on pretty suddenly. How do I know it's menopause, adrenal fatigue, or something worse? I hardly have the energy to get dressed."

"Anyone else develop severe joint pain, tendinitis, muscle weakness and muscle wasting from menopause? Estrogen helped but I got used to the estrogen and it came back. I've been to NAMS professionals and rheumatologists. I'm healthy in every way. I went from 20 pound curls to 3 pounds due to pain. It's the same with all arm muscle groups. I'm a PTA, my BF is a chiro and I still use a personal Trainer. It's not from overuse or poor form. Celebrex helps immensely but I can't be on that forever. I'm seeing another menopause specialist to see if my estrogen can be increased and stop this pain"

"I know it's been brought up before, but can we talk fatigue and muscle weakness? My legs are tired just going to my upstairs. All I want to do is sleep. What are others taking? I take biotin, b-12 and b complex, vitamin d, collagen and hrt. I was just reading about CoQ10. Anyone take this with good results? Any other recommendations? I want my energy back!"

Out of Nowhere: Menopause & Heart Palpitations

Terror took hold when my heart abruptly started racing. Panic surged as I fumbled for my pulse, confirming the frantic rhythm thrumming through my chest. Sometimes the pounding wasn't frantic, but a relentless, powerful beat that seemed to echo through my entire body. The fear of a hidden heart condition was paralyzing. Was a trip to the emergency room necessary? Thankfully, these online posts became my lifeline, dispelling the isolation and revealing a comforting truth: I wasn't alone.

"Anyone get heart palpitations where your heart feels like it's skipping beats you feel like you can't breathe it only lasts a few seconds but it's scary I been to the cardiologist he's done echocardiogram,ekg and I had a chest x-ray done i even had to wear a heart monitor for a month he says everything was normal sometimes it gets to where I wanna go to hospital but with in the past year I've been to the hospital 4 times and every test comes out normal."

"What does everyone do for their heart health? I'm still getting a racing heart , palpitations and flutters and some chest pains. But my doc thinks it's because of having no estrogen and a high fish. Tonight will be night 3 of double dosing on my current bhrt. If this is going to help, I sure wish it would kick in more quickly! I take magnesium glycinate and threonate along with nitric oxide. And I just started

eating and drinking beets to see if that would do anything for me.

Gosh, this is such a roller coaster ride."

"Hi, new here! For those of you who've experienced heart palpitations as a symptom, how many days did they last? Did they gradually go away or get less noticeable, or did you wake up one day and suddenly they were gone?

I'm 52 and in peri and that symptom started for me yesterday and I HATE it. It's so scary and disconcerting and I tend to catastrophize it thinking "Am I about to have a heart attack?" People say it's normal but it certainly doesn't FEEL normal!"

"Has anybody has issues with breathlessness and heart palpitations? For the last 10 months I've been struggling to lay flat at night because I can't breathe properly. Sometimes when I walk I can get a little breathless and also I feel like my heart tightens and just feels really strange. It's really hard to describe. I thought this was originally down to anxiety and being really worried about these more physical elements. My anxiety has started to get worse again. Then two days ago I downloaded a menopause app and they ask you to tick all symptoms. I was shocked to see breathlessness and heart palpitations on the list. I didn't know this could be linked to menopause. I've got a doctor's appointment now to discuss. Has anybody else had this? "

"Hi all, can you please explain your heart palpitations?
Yesterday my heart rate suddenly jumped to 120 and then bounced back to normal in less than two minutes. I felt slightly dizzy. I went to the ER two times for this and had a heart echo and everything was normal. I'm 41 and premenopausal "

The Symptom Spiral: Pre-Menopause and the Escalation of Anxiety

Armed with therapy, medication, and mindfulness techniques, I'd successfully managed my diagnosed Generalized Anxiety Disorder for years. Then, pre-menopause hit. The sudden onslaught of unfamiliar symptoms was terrifying. Were they something more sinister? My doctor's inconclusive answers only fueled my worry. The hormonal roller coaster added another layer of chaos, sending my anxiety skyrocketing. Tears became a constant companion, a helpless response to the emotional turmoil.

"My anxiety has gotten extreme! I don't want to be around ppl but I don't want to be alone either! I think I'm dying and something is wrong like I'm having a heart attack or I have cancer. I do have some health issues going on now but it's making my anxiety just unbearable...God please help me...I just can't anymore!"

"Really Really struggling with anxiety and fears of de@th to the point of not sleeping, not looking after myself and feeling genuinely terrible. I keep thinking it's my last day on earth. I have no motivation to do anything at all, can anyone recommend anything or have any of you been in this situation?
I've never been so rock bottom. Hopefully speaking with the gp tomorrow but he's going to say the same thing no doubt, antidepressants. Any advice please"

"Does anyone have issues with sleeplessness due to anxiety? How do you cope? Every night, around 4 am I wake up with a really bad anxiety attack and can't go back to sleep, and if I do, it is like 2 hours later and it is time to get up. It is so debilitating. I am exhausted most of the time. I have anxiety issues during the day as well but during the day they are manageable. I am so tired of it "

"Does anyone here deal with anxiety that feels like it just goes on all day long and all night long? And with it negative thoughts, moodiness, crying spurt, feeling like you are never going to make it through this? This is where I'm at and it's getting so old and now I'm getting so frustrated. I see a psychologist too. I Take Amberen, magnesium, vit c, vit d3 with k2, Coq10, quercetin, zinc, saffron and I just added levium. And I eat extremely healthy and it just feels like nothing gives for me. I feel so helpless and my family doesn't "get me." Now I feel like I have anxiety on top of menopause anxiety and it is just overwhelming me so *much. My family doesn't know what to say, what to do to help (all men) and so I feel like I'm doing this all alone."*

"How is a person supposed to date with this insane anxiety?? So much for a social life! Is anyone on Effexor? Wondering what kind of results you got from it. My dr said no to HRT and put me on this instead so I'm hoping for some good results. She said they have helped a lot of women."

From Scalp to Butt: The Mystery of the All-Over Itch

A maddening itch took hold, a relentless creeper that spread from my scalp to my butt. Ears, arms, legs – nowhere was spared. What triggered this sudden assault? Allergies? Body products gone rogue? The frustration was a match for the itch, fueling a simmering pot of irritability. I got the itch to read more posts on this symptom (pun intended).

"Help! Intense itching on back, neck and chest. No rash. Maybe a few little bumps. Does anyone use special lotions that's soothing and helps? I've tried allergy pills and it's not helping. Just came on suddenly. I didn't eat or use anything different."

"Hey everyone. So I've been having severe itching on my arms and legs when I start to sweat or get hot. It started last summer and has not stopped. My dermatologist prescribed me allergy meds but it doesn't work. He has no idea why my body does this. I've never had this problem before. Does anyone else go through severe itching from heat that takes a while to go away? Sometimes the itching feels like needles being stuck through my skin. Someone help me. I'm an outdoorsy person and love nature but can't go outside anymore due to the heat. Any ideas because I'm out of options."

"I thought I had the itching under control - it's back and worse than ever. Any advice please I have tried creams, been to the Dr and had prescription steroid cream but that's not working. Driving me mad. It's worse than the insomnia and night sweats"

"Ladies, I need your help! I have had itching all over my body from time to time and mostly at night but it hasn't been bad. Then last night I started itching around 8pm and kept getting worse as the night went on. It drove me insane, I was always scratching somewhere all night I, I got little sleep. I've never had it that bad before! Can you ladies please give me recommendations on a cream or lotions or anything else that has helped you if you have dealt with this same thing? Thank you!"

"Well, I have been to every sort of doctor about my skin itching on my arms and legs. Even had a food

allergy test, a waste of money. I have narrowed it down to Histamine Intolerance. Up all night scratching with hives and the list goes on. My only relief is putting ice packs on my arms. Everything I read points in that direction. Has anyone had any experience with this? I have to say this has been the most difficult, painful, emotional and exhausting 6 months of my life. Any advice would be greatly appreciated"

The Disappearing Spark: A Look at the Symptom of Low Libido in Menopause

Intimacy, a source of joy, became a chore. My body no longer seemed to respond the way it used to. A touch that once sent shivers down my spine now felt…ordinary. The spark, the excitement – they were fading, replaced by a puzzling indifference. The frustration was palpable, not just for myself, but for my partner. Was something wrong with me? Was I broken? Confusion and a feeling of loss settled in, leaving a heavy silence where laughter and passion once resided. These posts helped.

"I have absolutely NO libido at all. None. Zilch. To the point, the idea almost repulses me. It's wrecking my marriage. I was never like this until about a year or so ago when at the same time my period stopped for several months at a time then started back up etc. So I'm not in full menopause but probably getting close."

"I'm DESPERATE & at my wit's end...my libido was never really high, but it was there. As I've gotten older it's disappearing altogether. This upsets me A LOT because I have a wonderful, loving, and understanding husband of whom I want to show more affection. My first OB told me it was in my head and to force it until it became normal. Second was willing to put me on medication, but due to an autoimmune issue, side effects aren't worth the risk.

I've done every natural supplement, every tea, every food, exercise, etc. Nothing, not even a little. Has anyone ever tried a hypnotist for libido. It's a very serious question, I know I'll get some laughs, but I'm willing to try it, just want to see if anyone else has thought about this."

"Just a thought on loss of libido & vaginal atrophy: I think there are 2 TOTALLY different issues going on. The first is lack of libido: no interest in sex or just not being "in the mood." In that case I have usually just done it anyway, & I usually ended up enjoying it. But, since the atrophy got so bad, it's not just not being in the mood. The pain is ALMOST unbearable during sex & then very sore w/light blood for a couple days after. I end up using a "numbing gel" just to "get through it". I am on Premarin & have used at least a half dozen otc meds & nothing helps much. My doctor told me there was nothing else she could do for me . So far, twice a month is the most I can handle, which isn't nearly enough for hubby. Not sure how much more of this we can take"

"Hi ladies. I constantly see posts about libido and sex drives that have disappeared. There's obviously a theme going here. I'm right there with ya. I've been in meno for at least 3 years and have finally accepted it. So now what I wanna know is....does it ever return?? Has anybody had a comeback (even to some degree) after 'xyz' years? Or is this something for the history books that we'll be telling our grandkids, "I remember when I would..."?"

From Restful Nights to Restless Battles: Insomnia and Perimenopause

Sleep, once my reliable companion, became a distant memory. Perimenopause turned restful nights into a battle. Hot flashes jolted me awake, leaving me drenched in sweat. Chills followed close behind, a cruel reminder of the temperature fluctuations. But physical discomfort wasn't the only enemy. Anxiety, fueled by the uncertainty of it all, took root. How bad would it get? My mind churned, refusing to quiet. Agitation settled in, a relentless buzz that kept my body restless and my mind racing. Here's how other women described their insomnia symptoms.

"I know I have been on here before about my insomnia. I can't take it anymore. I think the lack of sleep is starting to catch up with me. I wake up shaky. I feel horrible. I am crying right now because I don't know how much more of this I can take. I can deal with everything else with this

menopause but this insomnia is killing me. Thank you lovely ladies for listening. Any suggestions on what to do and what actually helps some of you. I have Calm magnesium gummies but am afraid to take a maximum dose which is 4 because I do not want to overdose or take too much."

"I'm at my wits end with insomnia. I've tried everything to help me sleep. I often wake up every few hours to pee. I also have an extremely dry mouth which wakes me up. I've tried all the dry mouth stuff. I'm about ready to have a nervous breakdown or check into a mental health institute. I can't find a Dr to help with my hormonal imbalance. My progesterone is low and cortisol and dhea levels are extremely high. I'm working with a functional medicine doctor who is also a naturopath. She won't address my hormones. Just doing some supplements and food plans for detoxing the liver. I'm self employed and can't afford not to work. I don't know what else to do."

"Any recommendations for insomnia? I am having a terrible time staying asleep. I wake up with hot flashes and basically stay awake for the rest of the night. I have tried natural remedies of all kinds (melatonin, sleepy tea, estrogen night time, magnesium, Zzzquil pure z's, i meditate at night, keep room cool, exercise about 4 days a week, eat right, I even have resorted to Ambien, which I do not care for taking prescription meds, it knocks me out but makes me feel horrible the next day. Any

suggestions would be greatly appreciated because the lack of sleep is becoming unbearable."

"Hello ladies, any suggestions on serious insomnia? It has been ridiculous, and gotten worse than before. I even quit drinking coffee for two months now. I am pretty active during the day, but my heart rate goes super fast and makes me wide awake at night. I don't take a nap either. I would like to hear your suggestions. I am 54, I stopped my period 4 years ago completely. Thank you in advance for sharing your thoughts!"

My Menopause Weight Gain Woes

For years, I've rocked my curves – never skinny, but always comfortable in my own skin. By my forties, I'd figured out a routine: staying active kept my weight steady, and my belly, well, it matched the women in my family. Then, pre-menopause decided to join the party, and everything went haywire. Nothing I did seemed to make a difference. The pounds kept piling on, especially around my middle. It felt like I was constantly carrying a spare tire! Hunger was always especially for sugary carbs. It was like my body was craving a constant sugar rush. Okay, let's be honest, I do overeat sometimes, way more than I used to. Before menopause, I could control those cravings. Now, it's a whole new ball game. Is anyone else out there struggling with this perimenopause weight gain?

"Estradiol weight gain? Testosterone anyone? I gained 22 pounds in a short time, and my face looks

old, my belly hangs. I was so fit and young looking just 4 years ago . I've been on the estradiol patch for 4 years. I can't lose weight. Is it the estradiol? Can y'all please share your success stories with the hormones you take? I exercise almost daily."

"So this weight gain is NO JOKE! Just like, overnight! Oh here's an extra 20-25 lb's - good luck carrying that around UGH! I joined a gym in Jan and after 6 weeks developed Plantar Fasciitis..so painful to walk especially in the mornings. So needless to say, I have not done much of the gym since. Who does Keto? What about low-fat or Intermittent Fasting for the weight gain? Just trying to find something that works... along with alcohol LOL.. Not gonna lie - I do love a glass of wine or a cocktail on the weekends and everyone says that is deterring any weight loss. I am 1-1/2 years without period, so postmenopausal. Oh and I'm 57 in May (Yikes!) Up until menopause, I had never felt older than 35... love to go, go, go and I don't want to lose that. Thanks to all for listening"

"I'm having a hard time with weight gain. Every time I eat a little carb like a piece of bread or rice or pasta my stomach swells like a balloon and I gain 2-3 pounds right away. It's really tough being on a low carb diet eating vegetables and protein and nuts and seeds and a little fruit all the time. I just look at carbs and I gain weight. I can never lose any weight and I walk every day as well. What gives?"

"Ladies, reading so many posts about weight gain and the expansion of the middle tire, I've got an honest question to ask. I don't want to upset anybody but I'm curious. Do you think doctors in general steer too much away from any weight related? Would you have appreciated your doctor being honest with you at the start of your weight gain journey and would you have listened if they had told you how going through menopause would make weight gain more likely.
I am so saddened to read posts about how much excessive weight some of you want to lose and I'm slightly upset that physicians aren't more honest."

When PMS Gets Savage: My Battle with Perimenopause Phantom Cramps

Pre-menopause can be a wild ride! Forget the usual period pain – I was experiencing phantom period symptoms that were way worse than anything I dealt with before. These intense pelvic cramps wouldn't budge with my old ibuprofen routine. Heating pads became my best friend for hours on end, but the pain lingered. Convinced my period was just around the corner and relief would come, I was frustrated to find out this was a whole new ball game. That's when I turned to the internet and was lucky to read these posts.

"hi, I'm new to this group. I've been scanning through and i haven't seen anyone talk about phantom cramping? Does anyone get fake cramps & bloating then no blood? Also I'm starting to miss periods.. sometimes I get one and it's horrendous ! then next month no blood, but cramps for like 2 weeks. Hot flashes only before I "should" get a period, and itchy ants biting my skin all over, makes me crazy! Am I alone here? I really just want this to be over... I'm afraid I've got a long row to hoe, am I alone?"

"Been having period cramps for just over a week now with no blood. Not had a period since December. Sometimes it's enough to take painkillers and other times it's like a niggling uncomfortable sensation. Is it normal to have this without bleeding? My stomach is

also constantly bloated. I need a period to make it go away but it doesn't happen."

" It's now been almost 60 days since the first day of my last period. A few weeks ago, I thought my period was going to start. I had cramps, pms, all the usual symptoms but no period. I just had a video appointment with my doctor as I had been having some other symptoms I was concerned about. The doctor said that it was normal to have all the symptoms that a period was coming and then not have one. She said this could happen along with a lot of other symptoms (some of which I am also apparently having) as I progress through menopause. Has anyone else had all the telltale signs their period was going to start but no period?"

"Y'all. These invisible periods hurt way worse than a regular period. I am at the point where I think I'd rather have the mess than this amount of pain. Anyone else having this so intense like this?"

"Hi everyone, I'm new here. I'm having a strange issue and I was wondering if any of you have had a similar experience? I am 57 years old and it's been eight or nine years since my last period. I went through a horrible menopause. All the typical nightmare symptoms. I always started my period around the first of the month, this whole time I get tiny little cramps for about a day when my period would have started and then it would go away and

Why Can't Doctors Figure It Out? The Frustration of Misunderstood Menopause

My body started acting weird with a bunch of new problems. I went to the doctor about the nausea, and they tested me for celiac disease. The women's doctor suggested I exercise more for the aches and pains, but neither figured out the real reason. Feeling lost and alone, I started reading books and searching online. Finally, I found some answers and felt a little better about everything. But I was still mad. Why were so many women left on their own to figure this out? Shouldn't doctors know more about all the symptoms that come with menopause? Why do so many of us have to go through a bunch of tests and worry about serious diseases, just because doctors don't have all the information?

"I'm tired of seeing doctors that don't even want to address the hormone fluctuations as the reason for the severe depression and debilitating anxiety I have

been experiencing. I wasn't feeling this way until perimenopause hit so it seems to me common sense would tell a person it is hormone dysregulation. In conventional medicine: 1. Hormones are a one size fits all 2. Doctors say lab work is often inaccurate as hormones are in a constant state of fluctuation 3. Testosterone is not one of the hormones routinely used in standardized hormone therapy even though it is a hormone that women's ovaries and adrenal glands produce 4. All depression and anxiety are treated the same even if driven by hormones. So you are set up with a psychiatrist and given antidepressants and anti-anxiety medications (if you're lucky) and treatments like electric shock treatment are discussed when you have failed medication trials on several medications and are now diagnosed with "treatment resistant depression". How can we be living in the twenty-first century with so many modern discoveries yet we have not been able to figure out menopause? I know I am ranting just feeling extremely frustrated this morning. Thanks for listening."

"Male doctors.... I've had more luck with female ones.... all the female doctors and GYNs brush off symptoms, I hear you're too young, it's all in your heart. Etc etc.... my male GP yesterday said anytime my spotting goes too heavy or long just call and he will send a prescription over, and then threw out lets text xyz (all diff stuff) to see where levels are and what we can do.... like without me asking even!!!! I need to find a good GYN but all the places here are *mostly female and ive been to and just brushed it off.... I live in a super rural area.... feel like i'm figuring it out all on my own.... well, with my natural health specialist also...."*

"I've been to so many doctors and have had so many tests ran over the last 3 years because I have not felt well at all. Praise God nothing serious has shown up but the doctors/specialists can't find what is causing all the awful symptoms in my body. I recently had some blood work done to see if I was in menopause and it shows I am. Wondering if this could be the cause of some of my symptoms."

"Some doctors stick with what they learned in school and call it a day. Imagine you are in IT, a tech wizard!! You graduated 10, 20, 30, 40 years ago and since then you haven't bothered to keep up with the latest technology. You just keep doing the same old. Well eventually you won't be helping anyone because times have changed, technology has advanced and we want up to date qualified tech people to help us. Ladies, we need to realize that many doctors do this. They don't top up their knowledge along the way. Also, menopause is BARELY taught in med school. Unless they specialize. So please, pretty please, trust how you feel, pursue better health and get a feel for your docs knowledge and interest in helping you. I do understand that HRT is not for everyone but many of us are being told no for NO REASON other than our docs' lazy ignorance. Be well ladies"

Part 3: Lighting the Way: A Call for Broader Menopause Awareness

Menopause symptoms across cultures

Our understanding of menopause is stuck in a hot flash. It's time to shatter this narrow view and embrace the rich tapestry of this global experience. Menopause affects women from all walks of life, and its symptoms deserve a broader conversation. Let's move beyond the limited stereotype and acknowledge the full spectrum of physical and emotional changes women face. It's a chance to celebrate the diversity of menopause and ensure women everywhere have the support they need to navigate this important transition.

The study titled "Menopause across cultures: a review of the evidence" explored how women experience menopause in different cultures. Here's a summary of its key findings:

- **Menopausal symptoms are global:** Women around the world experience symptoms like hot flashes and vaginal dryness during menopause.
- **Symptom variations exist:** The frequency and severity of symptoms differ significantly across cultures.
- **Beyond hormones:** Social and cultural factors likely play a role alongside hormonal

changes in shaping a woman's menopause experience.

The study highlights variations in reported symptoms, but doesn't delve into specifics for every culture. However, it does mention some interesting trends:

- **Hot flashes:** Not as universally reported as previously thought. For instance, Japanese women experience them less frequently than those in North America.
- **Other symptoms:** Some cultures report different symptoms more prominently. For example, South Asian women might experience more body aches and urinary issues compared to hot flashes.

Beyond Bloodwork: Equipping Doctors for Menopause

The frustration with the medical system during menopause is a story many women share. Doctors and GPs often seem ill-equipped to handle the vast array of symptoms. Hot flashes might get a mention, but the fatigue, joint pain, and muscle weakness plaguing us often leave them scratching their heads. Instead of connecting these dots to the hormonal shifts of menopause, we get bombarded with unnecessary blood tests and scans, all while the root cause remains unaddressed. It's a dead end, leaving us with no treatment plan and a lingering sense of confusion.

HRT, a well-established therapy, often gets relegated to a "last resort" due to outdated beliefs about its risks. What many women crave is a doctor who sees menopause not as a scary unknown, but as a natural transition with manageable symptoms. We need a healthcare system where comprehensive education equips doctors to recognize the full spectrum of menopause and offer effective treatment options, including BHRT when appropriate.

Menopause in the Workplace: A Global Shift Towards Support

The tide is slowly turning for women experiencing menopause in the workplace. While many countries haven't implemented formal policies, a shift towards recognizing and supporting menopausal women is gaining momentum. In the UK, for instance, government inquiries have recommended the creation of menopause policies for workplaces, while companies like Vodafone have rolled out company-wide initiatives offering resources and support. This approach isn't limited to Europe. Major corporations like ASOS, a UK-based company with international reach, have implemented gender-neutral policies covering menopause alongside other major life events.

These changes acknowledge the diverse experiences women have during menopause and aim to create a more understanding and supportive work environment. Although progress is slow, a growing number of countries and companies are recognizing the need to address menopause in the workplace, paving the way for a future where women can navigate this natural transition without sacrificing their careers.

Nobody told me! The Silence That Left Me Unprepared for Menopause

In my family, nobody ever talked about menopause. With three sisters, three aunts, and three female cousins, that's a lot of women! Even periods weren't something we openly discussed. Menopause seemed like a distant future, so it never came up. My mom, who I'm super close to, never mentioned her experiences, leaving me completely unprepared when I started getting symptoms.

This silence about menopause is a big deal everywhere. Nobody talks about it, which makes women feel confused and scared about a natural life transition. If talking about periods is awkward, imagine how hard it is to talk about menopause! Sharing stories openly would have been a game-changer. It could have helped me feel prepared and supported instead of alone and confused.

And let's be honest, sometimes even younger people and men don't quite get it. They might think we're exaggerating or using menopause as an excuse. But trust me, hot flashes aren't exactly a picnic, and the other symptoms can be brutal. Menopause is a real medical change, not just something women make up!

In the absence of open communication, I found myself downplaying my symptoms around my husband and kids. Instead of saying I had internal tremors, I'd simply say I felt cold. Heart palpitations became headaches to avoid scaring them. The terrible jaw tightness and pain I endured, I disguised as migraines. It felt easier than explaining the complexities of menopause and facing potential disbelief or misunderstanding.

In conclusion, while this book dives into a vast array of common and uncommon symptoms, remember, menopause is a personal experience. Women can encounter a wide range of physical, emotional, and cognitive changes. If you experience a symptom not mentioned here, further exploration is encouraged. Researching online resources or talking to other women in similar stages can be helpful. Ultimately, trust your body and seek medical attention if a symptom is persistent or concerning.

References and resources

General Information:

- **The North American Menopause Society (NAMS)**: https://www.menopause.org/
    - Offers a wealth of information on various aspects of menopause, including symptoms, treatment options, healthy lifestyle choices, and a glossary of terms.
- **Office on Women's Health (OWH)**: https://www.womenshealth.gov/
    - Provides a comprehensive guide to menopause from the U.S. Department of Health and Human Services.
- **The Menopause Foundation of Canada**: https://menopausefoundationcanada.ca/
    - A Canadian resource focusing on education, advocacy, and empowering women through menopause.

Symptom Management:

- **The Mayo Clinic**: https://www.mayoclinic.org/diseases-conditions/hot-flashes/symptoms-causes/syc-20352790
    - Offers detailed information on various symptoms of menopause and management strategies.

Treatment Options:

- **The American College of Obstetricians and Gynecologists (ACOG)**: https://www.acog.org/
  - Provides information on different treatment options for menopause symptoms like hormone therapy, lifestyle changes, and complementary therapies.
- **National Center for Complementary and Integrative Health (NCCIH)**: https://www.nccih.nih.gov/health
  - Explores the use of complementary and integrative healthcare approaches for managing menopause symptoms.
- **Researchers review findings and clinical messages from the Women's Health Initiative 30 years after launch:** https://jamanetwork.com/journals/jama/fullarticle/195120
  - This article explores the WHI study's findings and how they've been interpreted over time, providing valuable context for considering hormone therapy as a potential menopause management option.

Cross-Cultural Perspectives:

- **PubMed Central - Menopause across cultures: a review of the evidence**: https://www.ncbi.nlm.nih.gov/pmc/articles/PMC6970345/ (This article reviews research on menopause symptoms across various cultures and highlights the importance of considering cultural factors)

Menopause in the Workplace:

- **Harvard Business Review - How Companies Can Support Employees Experiencing Menopause**: https://hbr.org/2024/01/how-companies-can-support-employees-experiencing-menopause
  - Discusses the impact of menopause on work performance and offers strategies for employers to create a more supportive workplace for women experiencing menopause.
- **The Menopause Charity - Workplace Menopause Leave: What it Looks Like and Why It Matters**: https://www.mindsethealth.com/matter/workplace-menopause-leave
  - Explores the concept of menopause leave and its potential benefits for both employees and employers.
- **Canadian Centre for Occupational Health and Safety (CCOHS) - Menopause in the Workplace**: https://www.ccohs.ca/oshanswers/psychosocial/menopause.html
  - Provides a Canadian perspective on the challenges of menopause in the workplace and offers resources for employers and employees.

Disclaimer: This list is not exhaustive and it's always recommended to consult with your healthcare provider for personalized advice and treatment options.

www.ingramcontent.com/pod-product-compliance
Lightning Source LLC
Chambersburg PA
CBHW051700250726

48653CB00007B/2760